THE GREAT PHYSICIAN'S R$_x$ FOR
7 WEEKS OF WELLNESS
SUCCESS GUIDE

THE GREAT PHYSICIAN'S

for

7 WEEKS OF WELLNESS

SUCCESS GUIDE

JORDAN RUBIN

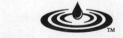

NELSON IMPACT
A Division of Thomas Nelson Publishers
Since 1798

www.thomasnelson.com

Copyright © 2006 Jordan S. Rubin

Published by Nelson Impact, a Division of Thomas Nelson, Inc., P.O. Box 141000, Nashville, Tennessee 37214.

Scripture quotations marked CEV are taken from the Contemporary English Version. Copyright © 1991 by the American Bible Society. Used by permission.

Scripture quotations marked NASB are taken from the New American Standard Bible, © 1960, 1977 by the Lockman Foundation.

Scripture quotations marked NIV are taken from the New International Version®. Copyright © 1973, 1978, 1984, International Bible Society. Used by permission of Zondervan. All rights reserved.

Scripture quotations marked NKJV are taken from the New King James Version. Copyright © 1979, 1980, 1982, Thomas Nelson, Inc.

ISBN 1-4185-0934-5

Printed in the United States of America.

05 06 07 08 09 RRD 5 4 3 2 1

CONTENTS

Preface   vii

Introduction: Offer Your Body as a Living Sacrifice   ix

Key # 1: Eat to Live   1

Key # 2: Supplement Your Diet with Whole Food   13
       Nutritionals, Living Nutrients, and Superfoods

Key # 3: Practice Advanced Hygiene   25

Key # 4: Condition Your Body with Exercise and Body Therapies   37

Key # 5: Reduce Toxins in Your Environment   51

Key # 6: Avoid Deadly Emotions   61

Key # 7: Live a Life of Prayer and Purpose   73

Video Curriculum Questions   93

About the Author   101

PREFACE

Dear Friend,

Not many years ago I found myself struggling with what was termed an "incurable" disease. After conventional and alternative health treatments failed, God revealed how His Word held the restorative health answers I was looking for. Ever since I recovered from my illness, I have had a passion and a commitment to help God's people reclaim their health and become better stewards of this valuable gift from Him.

My vision is that every one of the nation's leading TV programs, radio broadcasts, magazines, and newspapers would report scientific evidence showing that followers of Jesus are three, four, or even five times healthier than those who don't believe in Jesus—that Christians have fewer incidents of cancer, heart disease, diabetes, and obesity. Wouldn't it be awesome if God's people were so full of good health, so vibrant, that others would notice us from ten or twenty feet away and wonder what our secret is? What an opportunity to introduce them to the life-transforming power of the living God!

This vision may seem like a fantasy, but I believe it is a reality well within our reach. I am convinced that God's people can set the standard in health, and that is why I am presenting you with the 7 Weeks of Wellness program. The bottom line is this: If we want to effectively reach the world for the Lord, we need our health. If we take care of our bodies (God's temple) by following biblical principles confirmed by science, we each can extend the length and quality of our lives and better fulfill the great purposes God has for us.

This construction of the 7 Weeks of Wellness program is based on a biblical seven-week cycle—49 days of intentional health and wellness, with day 50 serving as both a day of celebration or jubilee and also as a continuation of the healthy foundation established during the initial 49-day period. In the book of Leviticus, God commands His people, "Seven weeks after you offer this bundle of grain, each family must bring another offering of new grain. Do this exactly fifty days later, which is the day following the seventh Sabbath" (Lev. 23:15–16 CEV).

This particular numbering of the days between Passover and Pentecost is referred to as the "counting of the omer" (literally the wave sheaf of barley— the first fruits) and signifies a period of passage from slavery to freedom and celebration. In this "omer count" lies special significance for Christians. We are God's "first fruits," offering ourselves to Him as living sacrifices—accounting for and numbering our days.

These seven-week cycles are celebrated as times of spiritual growth, and as we go through this 50-day adventure together, my prayer is that all of you can achieve greater health in body, mind, and spirit.

May God bless you as you begin your personal journey toward better health.

Jordan S. Rubin

Introduction

People who don't eat or live healthily are not thriving the way God wants them to. The 7 Weeks of Wellness program presented in this book is designed to help people recapture health and vitality that have been lost because of dietary and lifestyle choices.

Most people have one of two basic perspectives about their health:

1. Health = the absence of illness (the standard definition of health)
   - A person with this mentality says, "I don't have to do anything about my health *until* I get sick."
   - A reactive approach to health
   - A foolish perspective that reflects poor stewardship

2. Health = the presence of vibrancy (a new way of viewing health)
   - A person with this mentality says, "I need to *actively work* to maintain vibrant living."
   - A proactive approach to health
   - A wise perspective that reflects honorable stewardship

These two approaches to health summarize the core message of Proverbs: follow the path of the wise, and neglect the way of the fool. If you choose to be wise, you will follow seven practical daily steps to help you become proactive and strategic in your approach to vibrant living. This may be a harder path for you to travel, but in the end it will provide a longer and more abundant and honorable path for your life.

My core message of health is derived from two Scriptures:

Romans 12:1: "I urge you, brothers, in view of God's mercy, to offer your bodies as living sacrifices, holy and pleasing to God—this is your spiritual act of worship" (NIV). Are you presenting your physical body as a living sacrifice? Can you say, "This is the best I have, and I'm giving it to the Lord"?

Your body is a gift from God. Caring for a gift shows your reverence for the gift-giver and provides a way for you to worship and honor your Creator. "This is your spiritual act of worship" is not a request; it is a bold declaration that what you do with your life and your body must come from a desire to worship the Lord.

Genesis 1:26: "Let us make man in our image" (NIV). You were created in the image of God. Do you reflect His image? Do certain aspects of your health stifle God's image in your life?

By desiring to be a living sacrifice and by worshiping the Lord, you also recognize a sense of responsibility—stewardship. The fruits of stewardship can be grown only in the fertile soil of worship, so making conscious decisions in life to uphold and promote God's image will mean that you are choosing a life of stewardship. A life that proactively nurtures and strengthens God's image is a life He honors.

Good health goes well beyond the absence of disease in your life. We may not know how to articulate good health, but we know what it looks like. It's the father of four who works fifty hours a week but, after work, still has energy to go for bike rides with his family. It's a mother caring for herself and her family, whose children haven't missed a day of school in two and a half years. It's a grandparent who takes the grandkids to the park so Mom and Dad have some free time.

Good health is important to everyone at every age, and the 7 Weeks of Wellness program was written to help you reach your full and personal physical potential. God wants to use you; He needs you at your physical, spiritual, and mental/emotional best—and reaching this state requires effort. We are asked to offer ourselves as living sacrifices to the Lord—offering Him our lives in body, mind, and spirit.

Here are four reasons to offer your body as a living sacrifice to the Lord:

1. You'll enjoy long life and peace.

2. You'll live an abundant life.

3. You'll honor your family.

4. You'll honor God.

Food for Thought

- Romans 12:1 says, "I urge you, brothers, in view of God's mercy, to offer your bodies as living sacrifices, holy and pleasing to God—this is your spiritual act of worship" (NIV). And Genesis 1:26 says, "Let us make man in our image" (NIV). Do you consider yourself healthy?

- Can you currently say you are presenting your physical body as a living sacrifice to God?

- After reviewing this section, how do you think you can achieve overall optimal health from this point on?

- Is there an area you need to focus on most—body, mind, or spirit?

WHAT TO EXPECT

Our Goals with You

The 7 Weeks of Wellness program is designed to help you reach a higher level of health in body, mind, and spirit.

Body

- overcoming health issues
- sleeping and resting better
- increasing your overall level of health
- regaining lost energy
- losing weight (if needed)

Mind

- rethinking your ideas of health and wellness
- reducing stress and worry
- creating patterns of health for a lifetime

Spirit

- increasing closeness to God in your prayer life
- finding God's purpose for your life
- taking spiritual responsibility for your physical health

Your Goals

Take a minute to write down some goals you have during your 7 Weeks of Wellness.

Body:

_____

_____

_____

_____

_____

_____

Mind:

_____

_____

_____

_____

_____

Spirit:

_____

_____

_____

_____

_____

God's Plan for the Body, Mind, and Spirit

- God has offered an ideal "plan for living" so we can have overall optimal health in body, mind, and spirit.

- Overall health cannot be achieved by a singular approach; it must be approached in a holistic manner to include the body, mind, emotions, and spirit.

- Biblical principles serve as guidelines in every area of our lives, including diet, hygiene, exercise, mind-set, and so on, and they are still practical, relevant, and applicable today.

Practical Application of Timeless and Biblical Principles

- You will be guided in how to apply the seven keys to healthy living in your life.

- These seven keys will challenge you to give God the next seven weeks of your life to incorporate these timeless principles, allowing God to transform your health and your life.

- The Bible is an authoritative source on what we should and shouldn't eat and on how we should live. God, through his Son Jesus, has written a prescription for good health; it's up to us to fill that prescription every day of our lives.

Gradual Incorporation of Dietary and Lifestyle Keys

- You will be challenged to change or add elements of a healthy lifestyle over seven weeks, not overnight.

- The 7 Weeks of Wellness program incrementally incorporates both dietary and lifestyle elements to give you a complete health program.

- You gain momentum as you progress through the seven weeks, developing healthful dietary and lifestyle habits to last a lifetime.

- You will track your progress through each week and assess your implementation of change after each week.

- Depending on your health needs, you may focus more on some keys than on others. For instance, if you want to lose weight, you probably will focus more on food selection and exercise. Those who already maintain a healthy diet may focus more on supplements and body therapies. Use 7 Weeks of Wellness to customize your program.

Preparation for the 7 Weeks of Wellness

The 7 Weeks of Wellness program requires little preparation, but here are some helpful hints to make your experience as effective as possible.

- Purchase *The Great Physician's Rx for Health and Wellness* (if you have not already done so).

- Read ahead. Finish reading about each corresponding key in *The Great Physician's Rx for Health and Wellness* before trying to implement the key.

- Carefully read the protocol in *The Great Physician's Rx for Health and Wellness* before starting. Change is gradual, but it is helpful to be prepared for the change. For example, when the program recommends that you eat a healthy dinner, have a healthy option ready. Knowing the protocol ahead of time helps you stay on track and achieve greater results.

- For more information on the 7 Weeks of Wellness program, you may want to purchase the 7 Weeks of Wellness DVD (with Leader's Guide). Watch and listen to Jordan Rubin explain the details of his book *The Great Physician's Rx for Health and Wellness* and learn as he guides you through the Seven Weeks of Wellness. This is a great way to enhance your personal 7 Weeks of Wellness experience. Also, at the back of this guide are questions you can answer as you watch the video.

As you begin the 7 Weeks of Wellness program, please note that the program is designed to ease you into the changes gradually. At the beginning of each week, we offer a summary of the weekly key to health, as well as a helpful summary chart of the week's changes. Each day, we will give you the "New!" elements of the program. Please note that each day builds on the previous day and each week builds on the previous week's key. This means that in week 3, you will have changed your diet (week 1) and added supplements (week 2) and will be developing an advanced hygiene regimen. By the end of the program, you will have the 7 Weeks of Wellness integrated into the very fabric of your life and will have gained a comprehensive approach to health and wellness.

7 Weeks of Wellness is a 49-day program (seven weeks of seven days) that culminates on day 50, Jubilee Day, as a day of celebration and restoration. Day 50 also serves as the first day of the next "season" your life—a life shaped by offering yourself as a living sacrifice to the Lord and growing in the fullness of what He has for you in body, mind, and spirit.

The Counting of the Omer: Creating a Life of Worship and Stewardship

In the book of Leviticus, God says, "Seven weeks after you offer this bundle of grain, each family must bring another offering of new grain. Do this exactly fifty days later, which is the day following the seventh Sabbath" (Lev. 23:15–16 CEV).

God commands His people to "count" these days so they can honor and affirm the transforming work He has done in their lives. These days represent the time period between the first Passover in Egypt and the revelation of God at Mount Sinai. In other words, these days represent the journey of Israel from a people of slavery and bondage to a people of freedom and identity.

The counting of these days is referred to as the "counting of the omer," because the "omer" is the best section of the barley grain that God asked to be cut down and offered to Him at the beginning of barley harvest—the day following Passover. It was an intimate act of worship honoring what God had done in the past while looking forward to His provision in the future.

Like the Israelites, each day you are to count the omer, providing the best of who you are in an act of worship to Him. This is a daily acknowledgment of what He has done for you in the past, motivating you to be a good steward of your life as you move forward in faith. By taking life one day at a time, we can journey from slavery and bondage to freedom, identity, and purpose. Remember that each and every day of our lives is vital and builds into a lifetime of overcoming and celebration.

We are instructed to "count the omer" for 49 days until Pentecost arrives on day 50. This holds particular significance for followers of Christ. Christians are likened to the omer of the barley and are asked to offer themselves as sacrifices—living sacrifices—to God. Those who are in Christ and follow Him faithfully understand the journey from slavery to freedom. Therefore, we can do no less than live a life of daily worship and stewardship—of which health is an important part.

KEY #1

Eat to Live

Before you begin, read Key #1, "Eat to Live," in *The Great Physician's Rx for Health and Wellness.*

Food for Thought

- What do you believe constitutes a healthy diet and why?

_____

_____

_____

_____

- Describe "health."

_____

_____

_____

_____

- What foods are the most healthy and why?

_____

_____

_____

_____

- How much of what kinds of foods should you eat daily?

_____

_____

_____

_____

_____

- What foods do you avoid and why?

_____

_____

_____

_____

_____

- Outline a "normal" day of eating for you.

_____

_____

_____

_____

_____

- List some foods you will need to give up over the next week. If you can't think of any, check the "dirty dozen" (listed below).

_____

_____

_____

_____

- What do you hope to accomplish this week with your diet?

_____

_____

_____

_____

_____

Criteria for the Selection of Healthy Foods

There are three criteria we can use to identify the kinds of foods God intended us to eat (in a form that is healthy for the body):

1. *When God calls an item food.* "God said, 'I give you every seed-bearing plant on the face of the whole earth and every tree that has fruit with seed in it. They will be yours for food'" (Gen. 1:29 NIV); "[Y]ou will eat the plants of the field" (Gen. 3:18 NIV).

2. *When God brings items to His people as a gift.* "Also the food I provided for you—the fine flour, olive oil and honey I gave you to eat" (Ezek. 16:19).

3. *If Jesus ate or served an item.* "[H]e took the seven loaves and the fish, and when he had given thanks, he broke them and gave them to the disciples, and they in turn to the people" (Matt. 15: 36).

Additional Factors in a Healthy Diet

- *Organic foods.* The more convenient foods are, the less healthy and further away from God's design they are. Producing foods as cheaply as possible is the mantra of today's agribusiness, so *eat organic*—close to the natural source. Organic foods are minimally processed without artificial ingredients, preservatives, or irradiation to maintain the integrity of the food. It's all about quality. If you buy organic and if you shop for sustainably produced animal food, then you're purchasing some of the healthiest food you can buy, especially if it is properly prepared.

- *The Creator's basic food groups: proteins, fats, and carbohydrates.*

  Proteins. Proteins are required for the structure, function, and regulation of the body's cells, tissues, and organs and build body organs, muscles, nerves, and so on. Animal protein—chicken, beef, lamb, dairy, eggs, and so on—is the only complete protein source providing the eight essential amino acids.

  Fats. You have to eat the right fats—foods loaded with omega-3 polyunsaturated fats and monounsaturated (omega-9) fatty acids, as well as healthy saturated fats—found in a wide range of foods including salmon, lamb, and goat meat; goat's and sheep's milk and cheese; walnuts and olives; and butter and coconut oil.

  Carbohydrates. Carbohydrates are the starches and sugars produced by plant foods. Eat your carbohydrates fresh and unrefined—large amounts of vegetables and fruits, properly prepared grains, and small amounts of honey and other healthy sweeteners.

- *Top healing foods.* God has created some foods with wonderful healing properties. See the list and descriptions on pages 26–31 in *The Great Physician's Rx for Health and Wellness.*

- *The "dirty dozen."* These are some of the most popular and widespread food products and are the least healthy items you can put into your mouth.

  1. pork products
  2. shellfish and fish without fins and scales (catfish, shark, eel)
  3. hydrogenated oils (margarine, shortening, etc.)
  4. artificial sweeteners (aspartame, saccharin, sucralose)
  5. white flour
  6. white sugar
  7. soft drinks
  8. pasteurized, homogenized skim milk
  9. high-fructose corn syrup

10. hydrolyzed soy protein (imitation meat products)

11. artificial flavors and colors

12. excessive alcohol

When it comes to eating to live, we can use the acrostic EAT as our food guide. What foods are Extraordinary, Average, or Trouble? (For the full list, refer to pages 55–66 in *The Great Physician's Rx for Health and Wellness*.)

For more information on eating to live, see our free online course called "Eating to Live 101" at www.BiblicalHealthInstitute.com.

WEEK 1: EAT TO LIVE

Your Week at a Glance

Day	1	2	3	4	5	6	7
Upon Waking					Partial Fast	12–16 oz. water	12–16 oz. water
Breakfast					Partial Fast	Healthy	Healthy
Snack		Healthy	Healthy	Healthy	Partial Fast	Healthy	Healthy
Lunch			Healthy	Healthy	Partial Fast	Healthy	Healthy
Snack		Healthy	Healthy	Healthy	Partial Fast	Healthy	Healthy
Dinner	Healthy	Healthy	Healthy	Healthy	Healthy	Healthy	Healthy
Before Bed						8–12 oz. water	8–12 oz. water

You will begin the 7 Weeks of Wellness by changing your eating habits—slowly modifying your dietary patterns one meal at a time. To see the changes by day, refer to the chart above. By the end of the week, you will have three healthy meals, healthy snacks, and water in the morning and in the evening. You may want to drink your water in the evening an hour or so before bed if you have trouble sleeping through the night. Please refer to pages 69–73 in *The Great Physician's Rx for Health and Wellness* for the full details of the daily plan and for product recommendations. Continue to refer to this week's chart to monitor the daily regimen.

Helpful Hints

- Plan your meals ahead of time to maintain consistency throughout the seven weeks.

- Begin by slowly replacing the "dirty dozen" with more healthful alternatives.

Day 1

New!

Dinner

grilled chicken

green salad with red peppers, red onions, cucumbers, and carrots

baked sweet potato with butter

Daily Tip: This first step in healthy weight loss is to balance insulin. When carbohydrates are eaten in excess, or without protein and fat, insulin levels become imbalanced. Make sure to eat proteins, fats, non-starchy vegetables, and carbohydrates together.

Daily Notes:

_____

_____

_____

_____

_____

_____

_____

Day 2

New!

Snacks

    healthy whole food bar (see the *The Great Physician's Rx for Health and Wellness* Resource Guide, pages 329–30, for recommended products)

    piece of fruit

Daily Tip: Refined foods such as white flour and white rice are stripped of the fiber and nutrients that whole grains still possess. The first word on the label must be "whole."

Daily Notes:

_____

_____

_____

_____

_____

_____

_____

_____

Day 3

New!

Lunch

    Oriental Red Meat Salad (see appendix A of *The Great Physician's Rx for Health and Wellness,* page 266, for recipe)

    apple

Daily Tip: In the early 1800s the per capita consumption of sugar (sucrose) was about 12 pounds a year. Today in the United States, the per capita consumption of sugar is more than 150 pounds a year.

Daily Notes:

_____

_____

_____

_____

_____

_____

Day 4

Today, just focus on having a healthy lunch, dinner, and snacks.

Daily Tip: Consuming liquids such as herbal teas, nutritional soups and broths, naturally lacto-fermented beverages, and water is the healthiest way to supply our daily fluid needs. These fluids support, not inhibit, digestion.

Daily Notes:

_____

_____

_____

_____

_____

_____

Day 5 (Partial-Fast Day)

New!
Breakfast
   none (partial-fast day)

New!
Lunch
   none (partial-fast day)

New!

Snacks

   none (partial-fast day)

Daily Tip: Raw vegetable and fruit juices provide superior nutritional value. Consuming raw juices is the best means we have of getting all the vitamins, minerals, and enzymes needed to take care of our organs and tissues, our immune system, and all the vital functions of the body.

Daily Notes:

_____

_____

_____

_____

_____

_____

DAY 6

New!

Upon Waking

   12–16 ounces of water

New!

Breakfast

   Mexican Omelet (see appendix A of *The Great Physician's Rx for Health and Wellness,* page 305, for recipe)

   avocado

   salsa

   hot tea with honey (see *The Great Physician's Rx for Health and Wellness* Resource Guide, page 339, for recommended herbal tea blends)

New!

Before Bed

8–12 ounces of water or hot tea with honey

Daily Tip: Nitrites are used to cure bacon and other pork products. They protect the consumer from botulism, but unfortunately, nitrites convert to the potent carcinogen nitrosamine in the body.

Daily Notes:

_____

_____

_____

_____

_____

Day 7

There are no new changes. Focus on having three healthy meals and healthy snacks. See *The Great Physician's Rx for Health and Wellness* for meal recommendations in Appendix A, page 265.

Daily Tip: The principle of fasting is simple. When the intake of food is temporarily stopped, many systems of the body are given a break from the hard work of digestion. The extra energy the body gains gives it a chance to heal and restore itself, and the burning of stored calories gets rid of toxic substances stored in the body.

Daily Notes:

_____

_____

_____

_____

The Week in Review

- What was the most difficult food to give up and why?

_____

_____

_____

_____

_____

- What foods did you rediscover or discover for the first time?

_____

_____

_____

_____

_____

- Has your digestion improved or have you noticed any physical changes this week?

_____

_____

_____

_____

_____

- List any other positive changes you have noticed this week.

_____

_____

_____

_____

- Offer God a prayer of thanksgiving for the progress you made this week.

_____

_____

_____

_____

_____

_____

KEY #2

Supplement Your Diet with Whole Food Nutritionals, Living Nutrients, and Superfoods

Before you begin, read Key #2, "Supplement Your Diet with Whole Food Nutritionals, Living Nutrients, and Superfoods," in *The Great Physician's Rx for Health and Wellness.*

Food for Thought
- What comes to mind when you hear the word *supplements?*

_____

_____

_____

_____

_____

_____

- Have you ever taken a supplement before? If so, what was your experience like when

  (1) shopping for one?

_____

_____

_____

_____

_____

_____

(2) choosing one?

_____

_____

_____

_____

_____

_____

(3) staying consistent?

_____

_____

_____

_____

_____

_____

- Why would supplements be recommended even if you eat a healthy diet (Key #1)?

_____

_____

_____

_____

_____

_____

Food alone may not give us all the nutrition we need to keep our bodies working at a peak level. Every person is different, and we all have different nutritional needs based on age, gender, geographical location, access to foods, levels of stress, and so on. Therefore, taking nutritional supplements that meet a need or deficiency of the body and that are in a form that the body can utilize is a key to reaching your health potential.

RECOMMENDED SUPPLEMENTS

Whole Food Multivitamin/Mineral Supplement

Taking a multivitamin that is in the form of food, which complies with the second criterion for eating to live—eat food in a form that is healthy for the body—is highly recommended. Take "living" multivitamin tablets in whole food form, also known as homeostatic nutrients—vitamins and minerals that have been fermented with probiotic microorganisms and their enzymes. These multivitamins contain a broad array of antioxidants from fruits, vegetables, herbs, and spices, and they are a great form of "health insurance."

Omega-3 Cod-Liver Oil

Omega-3 cod-liver oil contains four nutrients that hardly any of us get enough of. These four nutrients are eicosapentaenoic acid (EPA), docosahexaenoic acid (DHA), vitamin A, and vitamin D. EPA and DHA are long-chain polyunsaturated fats known as omega-3 fatty acids, best found in cold-water fish, especially the golden oils extracted from the filleted livers of cod, as well as wild fish body oils. Supplementing with omega-3 cod-liver oil in liquid or capsule form will help to prevent bone deterioration in adults, improve cardiovascular and immune system function, and contribute to long life.

Fiber/Green Superfood Combination

The average American consumes less than the recommended three to five servings a day of "greens," and the most beneficial are the deep green, leafy vegetables. A nutritious whole food fiber/green superfood formula combines the dietary benefits of whole food fiber sources for healthy digestion and low-temperature vegetables and green foods. If you're looking for nutrition on the go before you leave the house for work in the morning, a glass of a fiber/green superfood powder mixed in water or juice or a handful of easy-to-swallow capsules provides convenient nutrition.

Probiotic/Enzyme Blend

In addition to the loss of enzymes from food processing, we've been sterilizing our soil for the last fifty to one hundred years with pesticides and herbicides, which has destroyed beneficial microorganisms. Supplementing with a combination of carbohydrate-digesting enzymes and beneficial microorganisms known as "probiotics" in a whole food base will aid the body in digesting carbohydrates such as those found in processed foods, beans, and cruciferous vegetables and will support healthy digestive function.

Remember: High-quality whole food nutritional supplements can make a big nutritional difference in our lives. However, keep in mind that the term *supplement* means "in addition to." Be sure to base your health plan on eating healthy, organic food, using supplements only to aid in your quest for a long and healthy life.

For more information on supplementing your diet, see our free online course called "Whole Food Nutrition Supplements 101" at www.Biblical HealthInstitute.com.

WEEK 2: SUPPLEMENT YOUR DIET

Your Week at a Glance

Day	8	9	10	11	12	13	14
Upon Waking		FG	FG	FG	FG	FG	FG
Breakfast	WFMV	WFMV	WFMV	WFMV	Partial Fast	WFMV, PEB	WFMV, PEB
Snack							
Lunch	WFMV	WFMV	WFMV	WFMV	Partial Fast	WFMV, PEB	WFMV, PEB
Snack							
Dinner	WFMV	WFMV	WFMV	WFMV, CL03	WFMV, CL03 PEB	WFMV, CL03 PEB	WFMV, CL03 PEB
Before Bed		FG	FG	FG	FG	FG	FG

Key:
> WFMV = whole food multivitamin
> FG = fiber/green superfood powder or capsule
> CLO3 = cod-liver oil/omega-3 complex
> PEB = probiotic/enzyme blend

This week will build on week 1, and you will continue to enjoy healthy meals and snacks as well as drinking plenty of water as part of your daily routine. The chart above shows the gradual integration of supplements each day. Please refer to pages 98–105 in *The Great Physician's Rx for Health and Wellness* for the full details of the daily plan and for product recommendations.

Helpful Hints
- You may want to buy a pill organizer and/or measure out your daily supplements in the morning.
- Do your best to remember to take your supplements. It may take extra time and special reminders, but eventually it will become part of your daily routine.

Day 8

New!
Breakfast
Supplements: Take one or two whole food multivitamin caplets (see *The Great Physician's Rx for Health and Wellness* Resource Guide, pages 345–46, for recommended brands).

New!
Lunch
Supplements: Take one or two whole food multivitamin caplets.

New!

Dinner

Supplements: Take one or two whole food multivitamin caplets.

Daily Tip: By definition, probiotics are living direct-fed microbials, or DFMs, that promote the growth of beneficial bacteria in the intestinal tract. These probiotics crowd out harmful bacteria, viruses, and yeasts.

Daily Notes:

_____

_____

_____

_____

_____

_____

DAY 9

New!

Upon Waking

Supplements: Take one serving of a fiber/green superfood combination (see the *The Great Physician's Rx for Health and Wellness* Resource Guide, page 347, for recommended brands) mixed in 12–16 ounces of water or raw vegetable juice or one serving of green superfood capsules.

New!

Before Bed

Supplements: Take two tablespoons or five caplets of green superfood in 12–16 ounces of water or raw vegetable juice.

Daily Tip: Digestive enzymes can be replenished in two ways: by eating raw, natural foods and by taking enzyme supplements.

Daily Notes:

_____

_____

_____

_____

_____

_____

DAY 10

Continue the regimen with no new changes today.

Daily Tip: Antioxidants are a broad group of compounds that destroy single oxygen molecules called free radicals, thereby protecting the body from oxidative damage to cells. They are essential to good health and are found naturally in a wide variety of foods and plants, including many fruits and vegetables.

Daily Notes:

_____

_____

_____

_____

_____

_____

DAY 11

New!

Dinner

Supplements: Take one or two whole food multivitamin caplets and 1–3 teaspoons or 3–9 caplets of high omega-3 cod-liver oil (see *The Great Physician's Rx for*

Health and Wellness Resource Guide, pages 345–47, for recommended brands). **Daily Tip:** Ideally, we should be eating plenty of fiber in the form of raw fruits, vegetables, and whole grains. It is important to supplement with a formula containing sources of fiber as well as other nutrients or herbs that we would not normally consume in our standard American diet.

Daily Notes:

_____

_____

_____

_____

_____

_____

_____

_____

Day 12 (Partial-Fast Day)

This is a partial-fast day. Please refer to this week's chart to see the changes that coincide with your fast.

Upon Waking
Supplements: Take one serving of a fiber/green superfood combination mixed in 12–16 ounces of water or raw vegetable juice.

Breakfast
none (partial-fast day)

Lunch
none (partial-fast day)

New!

Dinner

Supplements: Take one or two whole food multivitamin caplets, 1–3 teaspoons or 3–9 capsules of high omega-3 cod-liver oil, and one or two caplets of a probiotic/enzyme blend (see *The Great Physician's Rx for Health and Wellness* Resource Guide, pages 345–48, for recommended brands).

Before Bed

Supplements: Take one serving of a fiber/green superfood combination mixed in 12–16 ounces of water or raw vegetable juice.

Daily Tip: Food sources of omega-3 fatty acids important for cardiovascular health, reduction of inflammation, and proper brain development can be found in cod-liver oil, high omega-3/DHA eggs, salmon, flaxseed oil, and walnuts.

Daily Notes:

_____

_____

_____

_____

_____

_____

_____

_____

DAY 13

New!

Breakfast

Supplements: Take one serving of a fiber/green superfood combination mixed in 12–16 ounces of water or raw vegetable juice.

New!

Lunch

Supplements: Take one or two whole food multivitamin caplets and one or two caplets of a probiotic enzyme blend.

Daily Tip: The United States Department of Agriculture estimates that more than 90 percent of the U.S. population fails to eat the recommended 3–5 servings of vegetables each day. If you mix a couple of scoops of fiber/green superfood powder into a glass of water or juice or one serving of green superfood capsules, you will be consuming one of the most nutrient-dense foods on this green earth.

Daily Notes:

_____

_____

_____

_____

_____

_____

Day 14

Continue the regimen with no new changes today.

Daily Tip: Protein has a fat-burning effect on the body, reduces hunger, and helps preserve muscles as those pounds drop off. The healthy option is choosing whey protein powders from grass-fed, free-range cows; fermented soy protein; or protein powder made from goat's milk. These are foods that God created in a form that is healthy for the body.

Daily Notes:

_____
_____
_____
_____
_____
_____
_____
_____

The Week in Review
- Do you feel a difference in your health? (Remember that it takes time to feel the full health effects of a good diet and supplements.)

_____
_____
_____
_____
_____
_____
_____

- Is there one supplement you may benefit from more than the others?

_____
_____
_____
_____
_____
_____
_____

- What was the biggest challenge in adding supplements into your diet?

_____

_____

_____

_____

_____

_____

- What steps can you take to help you be more successful in this area?

_____

_____

_____

_____

_____

_____

_____

- Offer God a prayer of thanksgiving for the progress you made this week.

_____

_____

_____

_____

_____

_____

KEY #3

Practice Advanced Hygiene

Before you begin, read Key #3, "Practice Advanced Hygiene," in *The Great Physician's Rx for Health and Wellness.*

Food for Thought
- How would you define "advanced hygiene"?

_____
_____
_____
_____
_____
_____
_____
_____

- What do you think is the connection between hygiene and illness?

_____
_____
_____
_____
_____
_____
_____

- How many common areas (railings, shopping carts, doorknobs) do you touch per day?

_____

_____

_____

_____

_____

_____

- How often does your family pass around the same illness?

_____

_____

_____

_____

_____

Hygienic Highlights

- Germs don't fly; they hitchhike!
- Germs prefer to hitchhike (on the hands and under the fingernails) rather than fly through the air. Once germs are established on your hands and fingertips, it is only a matter of time before you rub your eyes, scratch your nose, stroke your ears, or touch your mouth— letting the germs in those portals of entry.
- Sections of Leviticus, Deuteronomy, and Numbers outline laws that protected Israelites from communicable diseases.
- Germs break down your immune system and make you more susceptible to health problems. You can help minimize germ infestations when you take key steps to guard yourself against attack, such as washing your hands and nails with a quality soap and dipping your head into a facial solution that cleanses your eyes and nasal passages.

Steps in Practicing Advanced Hygiene

- Dip both hands into a tub of semi-soft cleanser—to clean the fingertips, fingernails, and cuticles. Do this for 15–30 seconds. Rinse under running water.

- Do the facial dip: dunk your face into a basin of warm water with two drops of mineral-based facial solution to get rid of germs in the eyes and nose area. (It's like snorkeling in the sink!)

- Apply very diluted drops of hydrogen peroxide and minerals into the ears (30–60 seconds) to cleanse the ear canals.

- Brush your teeth with an essential oil tooth solution to cleanse the mouth of any unhealthy germs.

For more information on practicing advanced hygiene, see our free online course called "Advanced Hygiene 101" at www.BiblicalHealthInstitute.com.

WEEK 3: PRACTICE ADVANCED HYGIENE

Your Week at a Glance

Day	15	16	17	18	19	20	21
Upon Waking	AH	AH	AH	AH	AH	AH	AH
Breakfast							
Snack							
Lunch							
Snack							
Dinner							
Before Bed	AH	AH	AH	AH	AH	AH	AH

Key:

AH = advanced hygiene

This week incorporates advanced hygiene daily. However, each day incorporates more aspects of advanced hygiene. Please refer to pages 121–32 in *The Great Physician's Rx for Health and Wellness* for the full details of the daily plan and for product recommendations.

Helpful Hints

- Give yourself extended time to practice advanced hygiene in the morning and evening. It takes only 3 minutes, but if you are unfamiliar with the system, it may take longer.

- Watch the protocols closely. They look similar, but each day builds on the others.

DAY 15

New!

Upon Waking

Advanced hygiene: For hands and nails, jab fingers into semisoft soap four or five times, and lather hands with soap for 15 seconds, rubbing soap over cuticles and rinsing under water as warm as you can stand. Take another swab of semisoft soap into your hands and wash your face. (See *The Great Physician's Rx for Health and Wellness* Resource Guide, pages 349–50, for recommended advanced hygiene products.)

New!

Before Bed

Advanced hygiene: For hands and nails, jab fingers into semisoft soap four or five times, and lather hands with soap for 15 seconds, rubbing soap over cuticles and rinsing under water as warm as you can stand. Take another swab of semisoft soap into your hands and wash your face.

Daily Tip: Keep waterless sanitizers in your purse or wallet in case soap and water are not available in the public restroom. These towelettes, although not ideal, are better than nothing.

Daily Notes:

_____

_____

_____

_____

_____

_____

Day 16

New!

Upon Waking

Advanced hygiene: Fill basin or sink with water as warm as you can stand, and add 1–3 tablespoons of table salt and 1–3 eyedroppers of iodine-based mineral solution. Swirl water. Dunk face into water and open eyes, blinking repeatedly under water. (See *The Great Physician's Rx for Health and Wellness* Resource Guide, pages 349–50, for recommended advanced hygiene products.)

New!

Before Bed

Advanced hygiene: Fill basin or sink with water as warm as you can stand, and add 1–3 tablespoons of table salt and 1–3 eyedroppers of iodine-based mineral solution. Swirl water. Dunk face into water and open eyes, blinking repeatedly under water.

Daily Tip: You do not need scalding hot water when washing your hands. Using warm water is fine!

Daily Notes:

_____

_____

_____

_____

_____

_____

Day 17

There are no new elements of advanced hygiene today. Continue to use the hand soap and facial dip in the morning and in the evening.

Daily Tip: Upper respiratory infections represent 80 percent of visits to doctors' offices. Advanced hygiene can help reduce the number of upper respiratory infections you experience.

Daily Notes:

_____

_____

_____

_____

_____

_____

Day 18

New!

Upon Waking

Advanced hygiene: Fill basin or sink with water as warm as you can stand, and add 1–3 tablespoons of table salt and 1–3 drops of iodine-based mineral solution. Swirl water. Dunk face into water and open eyes, blinking repeatedly under water. Keep eyes open under water for 3 seconds. After cleaning your eyes, put your face back in the water, and close your mouth while blowing bubbles out of your nose.

New!

Before Bed

Advanced hygiene: Fill basin or sink with water as warm as you can stand, and add 1–3 tablespoons of table salt and 1–3 drops of iodine-based mineral solution. Swirl water. Dunk face into water and open eyes, blinking repeatedly underwater. Keep eyes open under water for 3 seconds. After cleaning your eyes, put your face back in the water, and close your mouth while blowing bubbles out of your nose.

Daily Tip: Don't forget to wipe your shopping cart with a sanitary wipe before shopping!

Daily Notes:

_____

_____

_____

_____

_____

_____

DAY 19 (PARTIAL-FAST DAY)

New!

Before Bed

Advanced hygiene: Fill basin or sink with water as warm as you can stand, and add 1–3 tablespoons of table salt and 1–3 drops of iodine-based mineral solution. Swirl water. Dunk face into water and open eyes, blinking repeatedly under water. Keep eyes open under water for 3 seconds. After cleaning your eyes, put your face back in the water, and close your mouth while blowing bubbles out of your nose. Come up from the water, and immerse your face in the water once again, gently taking water into your nostrils and expelling bubbles. Come up from the water, and blow your nose into a facial tissue.

Daily Tip: If you wear contacts, remember to wash your hands thoroughly before handling your contacts.

Daily Notes:

_____

_____

_____

_____

_____

_____

_____

DAY 20

New!

Upon Waking

Advanced hygiene: To cleanse the ears, use hydrogen peroxide and mineral-based ear drops, putting two or three drops into each ear and letting stand for 60 seconds. Tilt your head to expel the drops. (See *The Great Physician's Rx for Health and Wellness* Resource Guide, pages 349–50, for recommended advanced hygiene products.)

New!

Before Bed

Advanced hygiene: To cleanse the ears, use hydrogen peroxide and mineral-based ear drops, putting two or three drops into each ear and letting stand for 60 seconds. Tilt your head to expel the drops.

Daily Tip: Hand washing is considered the first line of defense for avoiding illnesses in children!

Daily Notes:

_____

_____

_____

_____

_____

_____

_____

DAY 21

New!

Upon Waking

Advanced hygiene: For the teeth, apply two or three drops of essential oil-based tooth drops to the toothbrush. This can be used to brush your teeth or added to existing toothpaste. After brushing your teeth, brush your tongue for 15 seconds. (See *The Great Physician's Rx for Health and Wellness* Resource Guide, page 349, for recommended advanced hygiene products.)

New!

Before Bed

Advanced hygiene: For the teeth, apply two or three drops of essential oil-based tooth drops to the toothbrush. This can be used to brush your teeth or added to existing toothpaste. After brushing your teeth, brush your tongue for 15 seconds.

Daily Tip: After flying in an airplane, practice advanced hygiene to cleanse your hands and nasal passages. This will help your body stay healthy and free of illness-causing bacteria often found in public places like aircrafts.

Daily Notes:

_____

_____

_____

_____

_____

_____

_____

The Week in Review

- Was it difficult to make advanced hygiene a part of your daily routine? Why or why not?

_____

_____

_____

_____

_____

_____

_____

- Which part of advanced hygiene is your favorite?

_____

_____

_____

_____

_____

_____

- Are you more conscious of hygiene after this week?

_____

_____

_____

_____

_____

_____

- Offer God a prayer of thanksgiving for the progress you made this week.

_____

_____

_____

_____

_____

_____

KEY #4

Condition Your Body with Exercise and Body Therapies

Before you begin, read Key #4, "Condition Your Body with Exercise and Body Therapies," in *The Great Physician's Rx for Health and Wellness.*

Food for Thought

- What are your top three most common reasons (or excuses!) for not exercising? How might you find a way to get around these reasons? Be specific.

_____

_____

_____

_____

_____

_____

_____

- What are the long-term implications if you eat well but do not exercise?

_____

_____

_____

_____

_____

_____

_____

- Define what you perceive "body therapies" to be and specifically how they can work into a health plan.

_____

_____

_____

_____

_____

_____

- Describe what you have been told about the health effects of direct sunlight.

_____

_____

_____

_____

_____

_____

- Describe your typical sleep patterns for a week—amount of sleep, sleep quality, and so on.

_____

_____

_____

_____

_____

_____

- What challenges do you see this week in beginning to incorporate exercise and body therapies into your lifestyle?

_____

_____

_____

_____

_____

_____

- What steps can you take to help make this week successful?

_____

_____

_____

_____

_____

Common Excuses for Not Exercising
- I'm too busy.
- I don't have the time.
- I don't have the energy.
- I can't get up that early.
- I'm too fat.
- It costs too much money to join a fitness club.
- It's too cold.
- It's too hot.
- It's been so long since I exercised.
- There's something good on TV.
- I can't get motivated.
- If I exercise, I'll eat too much.

Exercise is important for losing weight and feeling good, but it is also important for reducing the risk factors for:

- high blood pressure
- diabetes
- obesity and overweight
- high levels of triglycerides
- low levels of HDL (good cholesterol)

Key Concepts

The Great Physician's Rx for Health and Wellness covers a myriad of topics in the chapter on exercise and body therapies. Take a minute to review these concepts and the brief descriptions accompanying each one:

- *Functional fitness (purposeful training).* Functional fitness is exercise that trains movements and not specific muscles.
- *Hydrotherapy.* This type of therapy uses water to heal and soothe the body.
- *Aromatherapy.* This type of therapy involves the sense of smell and uses essential oils to relax, invigorate, and enhance mood.
- *Music therapy.* This type of therapy uses music to enhance mood and can improve cognitive performance.
- *Rest and sleep.* Most Americans don't get enough sleep or rest; sleep deficiency can cause health and emotional problems and affect several areas of your life.
- *Sunlight.* Contrary to common belief, sunlight is good for you.
- *Deep breathing.* This type of therapy involves breathing from the belly to relax and give the brain a high-octane oxygen boost.

For more information on conditioning your body with exercise and body therapies, see our free online course called "Exercise and Body Therapies 101" at www.BiblicalHealthInstitute.com.

Week 4: Condition Your Body with Exercise and Body Therapies

Your Week at a Glance

Day	22	23	24	25	26	27	28
Upon Waking	Exercise	Exercise/ DB, BT	Exercise/ DB, BT	Exercise/ DB, BT	Exercise/ DB, BT	Day of Rest	Exercise/ DB, BT
Breakfast							
Snack							
Lunch							
Snack							
Dinner							
Before Bed	Exercise	Exercise, BT	Exercise, BT, Sleep	Exercise, BT, Sleep	Exercise, BT, Sleep	Sleep	Exercise, BT, Sleep

Key:

DB = deep breathing

BT = body therapy

Week 4 builds on weeks 1 through 3 as you continue to eat a healthy diet, supplement your diet, and practice advanced hygiene. As you start week 4, you will see that exercise is recommended daily. Please refer to pages 164–72 in *The Great Physician's Rx for Health and Wellness* for the full details of the daily plan and for product recommendations. Note that the regimen intensity recommendations build daily. This gradual increase allows you to incorporate exercise into your life without a lot of discomfort, and each day will highlight the new exercise or body therapy. Remember, sleep is considered a body therapy.

Helpful Hints

- Starting an exercise routine can be challenging, especially if you haven't been exercising; starting slowly will help you ease into this area without pain.

- If you are trying to lose weight, more exercise will help speed up your metabolism and burn calories.

- If you experience soreness, don't give up! However, don't push yourself to the point of injury. (Consult a doctor if you have serious pain!) Most exercises will get easier with daily repetition. Many of the body therapies can help your body recover quickly.

- Stick with the body therapies. If you find one you like, repeat it. This is a program for your health, so feel free to customize.

- Be intentional about getting proper rest. Your body may experience some changes during this week. Resting your body and allowing it to heal, rest, and recover are vitally important to your success.

- Finally, enjoy this time. Take your walks with a family member or a friend. Enjoy outdoor activities. Try to create experiences to enjoy rather than "working out."

- Pray you will be successful. You can also pray while you exercise. The Lord is listening!

Day 22

New!

Upon Waking

Exercise: Perform functional fitness exercises for five minutes (one round of exercises is found in Key #4, pages 138–45).

New!

Before Bed

Exercise: Go for a walk outdoors.

Daily Tip: Many essential oils have antimicrobial properties. They do more than smell good!

Daily Notes:

_____

_____

_____

_____

_____

_____

_____

Day 23

New!

Upon Waking

Exercise/deep breathing: Perform functional fitness exercises for 5 minutes (one round of exercises is found in Key #4, pages 138–45) and do deep-breathing exercises for 5 minutes.

Body therapy: Take a hot and cold shower. After a normal shower, alternate 60 seconds of water as hot as you can stand it with 60 seconds of water as cold as you can stand it. Repeat cycle twice for a total of 4 minutes, finishing with cold.

New!

Before Bed

Body therapy: Spend 10 minutes listening to soothing music before you retire.

Daily Tip: Getting sun is a great way to help fight vitamin D deficiency.

Daily Notes:

_____

_____

_____

_____

_____

_____

DAY 24

New!

Upon Waking

Exercise/deep breathing: Perform functional fitness exercises for 10 minutes (two rounds of exercises are found in Key #4 of *The Great Physician's Rx for Health and Wellness*, pages 138–45), or spend 10 minutes on a mini trampoline, also known as a rebounder (see *The Great Physician's Rx for Health and Wellness* Resource Guide, page 351, for recommended products). Finish with 5 minutes of deep-breathing exercises.

Body therapy: Get 20 minutes of direct sunlight.

New!

Before Bed

Exercise: Go for a walk outdoors or participate in a favorite sport or recreational activity.

Body therapy: Take a warm bath for 15 minutes with one cup of Epsom salt added.

Sleep: Go to bed by 11:30 p.m.

Daily Tip: An Ohio State University study showed a possible link between music, exercise, and cognitive ability. Those who listened to music while exercising showed greater cognitive output.

Daily Notes:

_____

_____

_____

_____

_____

_____

DAY 25

New!

Upon Waking

Exercise/deep breathing: Perform functional fitness exercises for 15 minutes or spend 15 minutes (three rounds of exercises are found in Key #4 of *The Great Physician's Rx for Health and Wellness,* pages 138–45) on the rebounder. Finish with 5 minutes of deep-breathing exercises.

Body therapy: Take a hot and cold shower. After a normal shower, alternate 60 seconds of water as hot as you can stand it with 60 seconds of water as cold as you can stand it. Repeat cycle 3 times for a total of 6 minutes, finishing with cold.

New!

Before Bed

Body therapy: Spend 10 minutes listening to soothing music before you retire.

Sleep: Go to bed by 11:15 p.m.

Daily Tip: Watch a newborn breathe. Babies are natural "belly breathers." We can learn how deep breathing looks by observing babies!

Daily Notes:

_____

_____

_____

_____

_____

_____

_____

Day 26 (Partial-Fast Day)

New!

Upon Waking

Body therapy: Get 20 minutes of direct sunlight.

New!

Before Bed

Body therapy: Take a warm bath for 15 minutes with 8 drops of biblical essential oils added. (See *The Great Physician's Rx for Health and Wellness* Resource Guide, page 350, for recommended products.)

Sleep: Go to bed by 11:00 p.m.

Daily Tip: Hydrotherapy can be traced back to the ancient Romans.

Daily Notes:

_____

_____

_____

_____

_____

_____

_____

DAY 27 (DAY OF REST)

New!

Upon Waking

Exercise: none (day of rest)

Body therapy: none

New!

Before Bed

Exercise: none (day of rest)

Body therapy: none

Sleep: Go to bed by 11:00 p.m.

Daily Tip: Dr. Claude Lenfant, director of the National Heart Lung and Blood Institute in Washington, says, "Adequate sleep is associated with good health and performance, as well as fewer accidents—an even more critical issue when children reach adolescence and need to be aware of the dangers of drowsy driving."

Daily Notes:

_____

_____

_____

_____

_____

_____

_____

DAY 28

New!

Upon Waking

Body therapy: Take a hot and cold shower. After a normal shower, alternate 60 seconds of water as hot as you can stand it with 60 seconds of water as cold as you can stand it. Repeat cycle 4 times for a total of 8 minutes, finishing with cold.

New!

Before Bed

Body therapy: Spend 10 minutes listening to soothing music before you retire.

Sleep: Go to bed by 10:30 p.m.

Daily Tip: Have your evening meal early. Finish your evening meal by 6:00 or 6:30 p.m. so your body's digestive processes can be at rest when you go to bed.

Daily Notes:

_____

_____

_____

_____

_____

_____

_____

_____

The Week in Review

- Exercise is often the most difficult part of a lifestyle to make a habit. How successful were you in incorporating exercise and body therapies into your routine?

_____

_____

_____

_____

_____

_____

_____

_____

- Which exercise or body therapy did you find particularly helpful or fun to do?

_____

_____

_____

_____

_____

_____

- Did your sleep improve and/or did you feel more rested when going to bed earlier? (Note: The program will continue to challenge you to go to bed earlier. Refer to _The Great Physician's Rx for Health and Wellness_ for detailed protocols for exercise and body therapies throughout the program.)

_____

_____

_____

_____

_____

_____

- Offer God a prayer of thanksgiving for the progress you made this week.

_____

_____

_____

_____

_____

_____

KEY #5

Reduce Toxins in Your Environment

Before you begin, read Key #5, "Reduce Toxins in Your Environment," in *The Great Physician's Rx for Health and Wellness.*

Food for Thought

- Describe a typical day in the areas of your water usage (drinking, showering, bathing, etc.); the quality of the air you breathe; anything you put on your skin (cleansers, lotions, makeup, etc.); household cleaners you use.

_____

_____

_____

_____

_____

_____

- Name seven possible toxins you encounter daily. What can you do to eliminate these toxins? Be specific.

_____

_____

_____

_____

_____

_____

- Find a bottle of lotion, makeup packaging, and so on, and make a list of the ingredients in these products. Do a quick online search of those ingredients and jot down some observations about them.

_____

_____

_____

_____

_____

_____

Toxins come in many shapes, sizes, and forms, and when it comes to eliminating toxins in your environment, the reference is to toxins inside your home: the air you breathe, the water you drink, the lotions and cosmetics you put on your skin, the products you use to clean your home, and the toothpaste you dab on your toothbrush.

Make no mistake. Contaminants are everywhere. PCBs, dioxins, furans, metals, asbestos, organochlorine insecticides, phthalates, VOCs, and chlorine are widespread and can be hard to detect. To stay healthy, we must reduce the number of toxins we encounter. This will allow our immune systems to function more easily and effectively.

Here are some suggestions to reduce the number of toxins you encounter daily.

1. Purify your water (both drinking and bathing).

2. Never cook in plastic containers.

3. Purify your air with plants and/or an air purifier.

4. Use all-natural cleaning products.

5. Use natural cosmetics and personal hygiene products.

For more information on reducing toxins in your environment, see our free online course called "Reducing Toxins 101" at www.BiblicalHealthInstitute.com.

Week 5: Reduce Toxins in Your Environment

Your Week at a Glance

Day	29	30	31	32	33	34	35
Upon Waking	RT	RT	RT	RT	RT	RT	RT
Breakfast							
Snack							
Lunch							
Snack							
Dinner							
Before Bed							

Key:

RT = reduce toxins

You have only three more weeks until your completion of the 7 Weeks of Wellness! Continue to build on the previous four weeks and make time this week to reduce toxins. As you can see, every day this week, we will try to reduce toxins. Each day is a little different, so refer to pages 193–201 in *The Great Physician's Rx for Health and Wellness* for the full details of this week's regimen and for product recommendations.

Helpful Hints

- Eliminating toxins is an ongoing process, so approach this week with a long term outlook. You will always need to be aware of toxins.

- Change at a pace that you can afford. If you can't afford to throw out all your cosmetics or hygiene products, just replace them with healthy alternatives when they run out. This will help you avoid an up-front "hit" in expenses.

- Don't be afraid to let out warm or cool air when opening the windows. Your heater or air conditioner will be able to catch up.

- Open your windows while exercising, especially if it is cool outside. You can accomplish two tasks at once.

Day 29

New!

Upon Waking

Reduce toxins: Open windows for one hour today. Make a plan to change air-conditioning or heating filters more regularly.

Daily Tip: Test your water. A pool test kit can be purchased and easily put to use to test the levels of chlorine in your city water. In most cases the amount of chlorine in the water you drink and bathe in is above the safe level for a swimming pool.

Daily Notes:

_____

_____

_____

_____

_____

_____

_____

_____

_____

Day 30

New!

Upon Waking

Reduce toxins: Open windows for one hour today. Purchase three houseplants and place them in your living room and dining area.

Daily Tip: *Organic Style* magazine cited a study of children who ate only organic produce; these children had one-sixth the level of pesticides in their bodies compared with children who consumed conventionally grown fruits and vegetables.

Daily Notes:

_____

_____

_____

_____

_____

_____

_____

_____

DAY 31

New!

Upon Waking

Reduce toxins: Open windows for one hour today. Purchase and install carbon-block shower filters for each shower in your home (if you're on city water). (See *The Great Physician's Rx for Health and Wellness* Resource Guide, page 354, for recommended products.)

Daily Tip: You should check and change the filters on your air-conditioning and heating units every month or so. This will result in much cleaner air flowing through your home.

Daily Notes:

_____

_____

_____

_____

_____

_____

_____

_____

DAY 32

New!

Upon Waking

Reduce toxins: Open windows for one hour today. Use natural soap and natural skin and body care products (shower gel, body creams, etc.). (See *The Great Physician's Rx for Health and Wellness* Resource Guide, pages 351–53, for recommended products.)

Daily Tip: One of the leading causes of death among children is the ingestion of cleaning products. Take the time to either get locks on your cabinets or replace your dangerous chemical cleaning products with natural cleaners.

Daily Notes:

_____

_____

_____

_____

_____

_____

_____

DAY 33 (PARTIAL-FAST DAY)

New!

Upon Waking

Reduce toxins: Open windows for one hour today. Use natural soap and natural skin and body care products (shower gel, body creams, etc.). Purchase and use natural facial care products.

Daily Tip: There are many soap-based cleaning products that will cause no harm if accidentally ingested. Vinegar is another safe alternative.

Daily Notes:

_____

_____

_____

_____

_____

_____

_____

DAY 34 (DAY OF REST)

New!

Upon Waking

Reduce toxins: Open windows for one hour today. Use natural soap and natural skin and body care products (shower gel, body creams, etc.). Use natural facial care products. Purchase and use natural toothpaste. (See *The Great Physician's Rx for Health and Wellness* Resource Guide, pages 352–53, for recommended products.)

Daily Tip: Get plenty of fresh air. If you are in an office and are unable to open the windows, try stepping outside for a breath of fresh air during your morning and afternoon breaks.

Daily Notes:

_____

_____

_____

_____

_____

_____

_____

_____

DAY 35

New!

Upon Waking

Reduce toxins: Open windows for one hour today. Use natural soap and natural skin and body care products (shower gel, body creams, etc.). Use natural facial care products. Use natural toothpaste. Purchase and use natural hair care products, such as shampoo, conditioner, gel, mousse, and hair spray. (See *The Great Physician's Rx for Health and Wellness* Resource Guide, pages 351–53, for recommended products.)

Daily Tip: The people of Israel were warned of the toxicity of mildew in their clothes and homes in Leviticus 13–14. It was something they were supposed to take seriously.

Daily Notes:

_____

_____

_____

_____

_____

_____

The Week in Review
- What changes did you notice in the air quality of your home?

_____

_____

_____

_____

_____

_____

_____

- How has this week changed your outlook on toxins?

_____

_____

_____

_____

_____

_____

- How did your body react to the natural skin and hair care products you tried this week? Note the changes and write them down.

_____

_____

_____

_____

_____

_____

- Plan steps to continue to eliminate toxins in these categories: water quality (drinking and bathing), household air quality, health and beauty.

_____

_____

_____

_____

_____

_____

- Start a savings account to save for some of the items you will need in the future. Save $5 a week and put it toward household plants, an air purifier, or new cookware. You are building habits for a lifetime, so set some goals to keep improving your health.

_____

_____

_____

_____

_____

_____

- Offer God a prayer of thanksgiving for the progress you made this week.

_____

_____

_____

_____

_____

_____

KEY #6

Avoid Deadly Emotions

Before you begin, read Key #6, "Avoid Deadly Emotions," in *The Great Physician's Rx for Health and Wellness*.

Food for Thought
- What specific situations cause a negative emotional response or negative thoughts in you? Be specific. How often do these situations occur?

_____

_____

_____

_____

_____

_____

- Make a list of the top five most important things in your life and explain why they are the most important to you. Then make a list of the five things that are least important in your life and explain why they are less significant to you.

_____

_____

_____

_____

_____

- Give a working definition of what it means to "respond" to a situation instead of "reacting" to a situation. Give an example.

  _____

  _____

  _____

  _____

  _____

  _____

  _____

- What are some emotions you can improve this week? Think of three ways you can help avoid these emotions.

  _____

  _____

  _____

  _____

  _____

  _____

- Make a list of the people in your life who need your forgiveness and the things for which you need to forgive them. Use this week to begin the process of forgiveness.

  _____

  _____

  _____

  _____

  _____

  _____

Deadly emotions lurk within each of us, ready to come to the surface at even the slightest daily prompting—a rough interaction with a family member or friend; an angry remark from a colleague at work; a clerk in a store who is less than professional in his or her interactions with you; hostile drivers on the interstate (or just about anywhere); or even your own "bad attitude" you woke up with! We need to get a handle on these emotions before they affect our joy and maybe our health.

Situations like these are part of being human, but we don't have to subject our health to the consequences of our deadly emotions. When we let our emotions take control, our bodies respond accordingly. For instance, hostile or angry situations cause the body's production of a hormone, cortisol, to run rampant in the body.

When this happens, blood vessels constrict and divert the flow of blood from leisurely bodily processes like digestion to quick-acting muscles in the arms and legs. The heart races to keep up and a heightened sense of alertness causes all sorts of anxieties. When this response happens repeatedly, the body begins to wear down. To avoid this wear and tear, we need to get a handle on these deadly emotions before they adversely affect our joy and maybe our health. When we get frustrated and harbor resentment and nurse grudges, our over-stimulated bodies produce the same toxins as if we binged on the worst junk food.

Not only can these negative emotions affect us physically, they can also affect us relationally with our family, our friends, our co-workers, and even our relationship with God. The results can cause a constant state of unhealthy stress or anger that eventually leads to arguments, depression, or compromised health.

Anger, acrimony, apprehension, agitation, anxiety, and alarm can be deadly, and when you experience any of these feelings—whether "justified" or not— the immune system becomes stressed. This kind of stress is a key source for a variety of ills including hypertension, headaches, hormonal imbalances, and elevated heartbeat. It is becoming more and more apparent to researchers that emotions are powerful forces within the human mind that clearly affect the body as well as the soul.

Why wait until your relationships, health, and joy of life are jeopardized until you choose to live the way you want to live—emotionally whole and content? Success in this area means that we need to control our emotions rather than have our emotions control us. We need to *respond* (thinking through and processing how we will act—having our raw emotions take a backseat) instead of *react* (acting without thinking—giving our raw emotions full reign) to what happens in our lives.

We need to ask ourselves about almost everything we encounter, "Is this worth it—really? Does this circumstance warrant this reaction or response from me?" The fact is that most, if not all, circumstances do not warrant a "raw," emotionally charged reaction. There is time to put our emotions on the back burner and respond to a situation rather than react to it.

Controlling Negative Emotions

How can we help to control negative emotions? By dealing with them as quickly as possible. If you have an argument with someone, make amends as soon as you can, or give yourself a "time-out"—enough time to refocus and collect your thoughts, to respond instead of reacting, and to calm down and breathe deeply, reminding yourself that this may not really be worth losing your joy. Letting go of anger and other negative emotions quickly means swallowing your pride and saying, "This isn't worth it."

Forgiveness

There is another negative emotion that God calls a sin, causes great bodily harm, and shortens one's life span—an unforgiving heart. Going through life without forgiving those who hurt you is like running a marathon with a fifty-pound weight vest on. It slows you down, wears you out, and can cause you to falter in running the race. By allowing anger and unforgiveness to take root and fester, a heart can become hardened by a constant state of anxiety. Remember: No matter how badly you have been hurt, unforgiveness will cause your health to suffer and will, more importantly, separate you from your heavenly Father.

Just because you forgive others doesn't mean that you will forget the hurt they caused you. However, you can be confident that God wants you to deal with your emotions so that you can lead a much healthier life on behalf of the Kingdom.

Strategy: Live in a State of Forgiveness

Because we live in an imperfect world filled with imperfect people, we are going to have to forgive frequently—everything from minor spills to major offenses. Choose to live in a state of forgiveness. Ongoing forgiveness keeps deadly emotions from building up.

For more information on avoiding deadly emotions, see our free online course called "Emotional Health 101" at www.BiblicalHealthInstitute.com.

WEEK 6: AVOID DEADLY EMOTIONS

Your Week at a Glance

Day	22	23	24	25	26	27	28
Upon Waking	EH	EH	EH	EH	EH	EH	EH
Breakfast							
Snack							
Lunch							
Snack							
Dinner							
Before Bed		EH	EH	EH	EH	EH	EH

Key:

EH = emotional health

With two weeks left in the 7 Weeks of Wellness, the focus changes to emotional health, but do not lose focus on physical health. Use this week to take steps toward health in body, mind, and spirit. Please refer to pages 217–27 in *The Great Physician's Rx for Health and Wellness* for the full details of this week's regimen.

Helpful Hints

- Decide *now* not to let deadly emotions take control of your life. Rehearse how you will appropriately respond (and not react) to situations that normally evoke negative emotions.

- Consider all you have been forgiven for—by others and by God—and decide to offer a forgiving spirit to others (with no strings attached).

- Look for opportunities to offer compassion to others and to forget offenses; remember to laugh more and to enjoy life!

- Since we live in an imperfect world with imperfect people, forgiveness and management of deadly emotions are daily (and sometimes moment-by-moment) habits you will use your entire life.

Day 36

New!

Upon Waking

Emotional health: When you face a circumstance that would usually cause you to worry, repeat the following: "Lord, I trust You. I cast my cares upon You, and I believe that You're going to take care of [insert your current situation]." Confess this throughout the day whenever you think about your circumstance.

Daily Tip: Get a handle on deadly emotions before they adversely affect your joy and health.

Daily Notes:

_____

_____

_____

_____

_____

_____

_____

Day 37

New!

Before Bed

Emotional health: Ask the Lord to bring to your mind someone you need to forgive. Take out a sheet of paper and write the person's name at the top. Try to remember each specific action that person did against you that brought you pain. Write down the following: "I forgive [insert person's name] for [insert the action he or she did against you]." After you fill up the paper, tear it up or burn it, and ask God to give you the strength to truly forgive that person.

Daily Tip: Send a note to someone special and tell them how much you appreciate them.

Daily Notes:

_____
_____
_____
_____
_____
_____
_____
_____

Day 38

Continue to cast your worries upon the Lord and to practice forgiveness in all situations. See *The Great Physician's Rx for Health and Wellness* or days 36 and 37 in this guide for exact protocols.

Daily Tip: Let go of pride and anger and say, "This isn't worth it."

Daily Notes:

_____

_____

_____

_____

_____

_____

_____

DAY 39

Continue to cast your worries upon the Lord and to practice forgiveness in all situations. See *The Great Physician's Rx for Health and Wellness* or days 36 and 37 in this guide for exact protocols.

Daily Tip: Spend a day riding in the "slow lane" on the highway. It will be a lesson in patience. It will also help you begin learning how to slow down.

Daily Notes:

_____

_____

_____

_____

_____

_____

_____

DAY 40 (PARTIAL-FAST DAY)

Continue to cast your worries upon the Lord and to practice forgiveness in all situations. See *The Great Physician's Rx for Health and Wellness* or days 36 and 37 in this guide for exact protocols.

Daily Tip: It takes no effort to be unforgiving, but it can take life and health from you.

Daily Notes:

_____

_____

_____

_____

_____

_____

_____

Day 41 (Day of Rest)

Continue to cast your worries upon the Lord and to practice forgiveness in all situations. See *The Great Physician's Rx for Health and Wellness* or days 36 and 37 in this guide for exact protocols.

Daily Tip: Smile—even if you have to force yourself! Eventually, you will be smiling because you want to.

Daily Notes:

_____

_____

_____

_____

_____

_____

_____

Day 42

Continue to cast your worries upon the Lord and to practice forgiveness in all situations. See *The Great Physician's Rx for Health and Wellness* or days 36 and 37 in this guide for exact protocols.

Daily Tip: Regularly tell your family you love them! Watch their reactions, especially if you don't normally say "I love you" often.

Daily Notes:

_____

_____

_____

_____

_____

_____

_____

_____

_____

The Week in Review
- How have you grown in the area of forgiveness?

_____

_____

_____

_____

_____

_____

_____

_____

_____

_____

_____

- How have your relationships with others improved this week?

_____

_____

_____

_____

_____

_____

_____

- What steps might you need to take to continue growing in the area of emotional health?

_____

_____

_____

_____

_____

_____

_____

- Offer God a prayer of thanksgiving for the progress you made this week.

_____

_____

_____

_____

_____

_____

_____

KEY #7

Live a Life of Prayer and Purpose

Before you begin, read Key #7, "Live a Life of Prayer and Purpose," in *The Great Physician's Rx for Health and Wellness.*

Food for Thought

- How can you incorporate prayer and purpose into your current circumstance? (You may want to pray and consider this question for a while before answering.)

_____

_____

_____

_____

_____

- Describe your relationship with God, and then give a working definition of prayer, describing a typical week and your "prayer pattern" with God. Give specific examples of your requests, your thoughts, and your dialogue with God.

_____

_____

_____

_____

_____

- Describe what you believe your life purpose to be, giving specific examples of what you do to fulfill that purpose.

_____

_____

_____

_____

_____

_____

_____

- Create a list of your top three talents and areas of giftedness—areas that are natural strengths for you that give you great satisfaction (and are very productive) when you engage them—and describe _how_ and _where_ you use them. Be specific.

_____

_____

_____

_____

_____

_____

_____

Prayer

Prayer is the foundation of a healthy life, linking your mind, body, and spirit to God. It is two-way communication with our Creator who built us for specifically for relationships with one another and with Him. Prayer is the tool by which we stay plugged-in to God. There is power in prayer, and the greatest source of power and strength resides in talking with the One who made us.

Prayer is not a formality and it is not about religion; it is about relationship. Because we are His children, we can talk to God anytime, anywhere, and for any reason. He is always there to listen, and He always has our best interests at heart.

In living a healthy, purpose-filled life, prayer is the most powerful tool we possess because it connects the entirety of who we are in mind, body, and spirit to God. Through prayer, God can take away our guilt, shame, bitterness, anger, unforgiveness, and can give us a brand new start in life.

Talking to God in prayer is foundational for health and has the potential to make us whole. After all, God's love and grace are the greatest foods for the soul. We need and crave intimate communion with God—to learn more about Him, to find our purpose, and to stay in a healthy relationship with Him!

Prayer Pattern and Fitness

Developing fitness in prayer is like developing physical fitness. In order to develop it, you will need to be diligent and intentional or it just won't happen. Without some sort of routine, you could get into a habit of talking to God only when you need Him to do something for you right away. That is no basis for a prayer relationship with God! Prayer is ongoing, personal, and requires a designated time. It does not just automatically happen; you have to plan time with God.

To be in a truly intimate, prayerful relationship with God, take the time to nurture your relationship with Him. Incorporate prayer into your daily life—thanking Him for how He has worked in your life, for who He is and for all He means to you. Gaining prayer fitness means daily communing with and living out the wonderfully intimate relationship and purpose with the loving Creator of the universe. Prayer also confirms your purpose in life and gives you the perseverance to complete that purpose, so be sure to seal all you do with the power of prayer.

Purpose

If you are not living a life of purpose, then you are like a lamp that is not plugged into the power source. No matter how hard you may try, you cannot do anything to brighten a dark room. God never intended for you to go through your life that way! He wants us to clearly know our purpose in life and to be about it. He knows that if we have no purpose in life, then we can become self-centered, self-serving, and spiritually immature.

You may not be exactly sure what your life's purpose is, but you can know that you were definitely created for a purpose. If you have not found your purpose yet, then search your heart and ask yourself these questions: *What makes you feel alive? What do you love to do? What are your personal strengths and skills? What are your values, beliefs, and philosophies? What are you passionate about?*

If you can pinpoint your passions and your natural talents, you will uncover your purpose. Keep in mind that God gives us different desires, different dreams, and different talents for a reason—to fulfill our purpose during our stay on Earth. A sense of purpose or mission gives our lives meaning and helps us to face each day with enthusiasm, focus, and determination. When we know our purpose, we know the importance of each day and understand how we should best spend our time, energy, and talents.

Find your purpose and then live it in your life, your family, your church, your organization, your community, and your region.

For more information on living a life of prayer and purpose, see our free online course called "Prayer and Purpose 101" at www.BiblicalHealthInstitute.com.

WEEK 7: LIVE A LIFE OF PRAYER AND PURPOSE

Your Week at a Glance

Day	43	44	45	46	47	48	49
Upon Waking	Prayer, Purpose	Prayer, Purpose	Prayer, Purpose	Prayer, Purpose	Prayer, Purpose	Prayer, Purpose	Prayer, Purpose
Breakfast							
Snack							
Lunch							
Snack							
Dinner							
Before Bed	Prayer, Purpose	Prayer, Purpose	Prayer, Purpose	Prayer, Purpose	Prayer, Purpose	Prayer, Purpose	Prayer, Purpose

This is the final week of the Seven Weeks of Wellness. Prayer and purpose are this week's focus. Please take this week to give thanks to God for what He has done in your life the past six weeks. Please refer to pages 246–64 in *The Great Physician's Rx for Health and Wellness* for the full details of this week's regimen.

Helpful Hints

- Prayer is communication with God and is founded on a strong relationship with Him. Talk with Him often, as you would with a trusted, longtime friend. He loves you and wants to be a part of your life.

- Develop a routine for prayer, just as you would for exercise. Since schedules vary, choose a realistic time for prayer that works for you.

- Determine which activities in your life are essential and which ones are not essential. Generally, activities that are essential (and that only you can do or have to be a part of) are those in line with your purpose.

- Knowing and acting on your purpose gives meaning, simplification, focus, motivation, and eternal impact to your life.

Day 43

New!

Upon Waking

Prayer: Thank God because this is the day that the Lord has made. Rejoice and be glad in it. Thank Him for the breath in your lungs and the life in your body. Pray and confess the following Scripture out loud:

> *Our Father in heaven,*
> *Hallowed be Your name.*
> *Your kingdom come.*
> *Your will be done*
> *On earth as it is in heaven.*
> *Give us this day our daily bread.*
> *And forgive us our debts,*
> *As we forgive our debtors.*
> *And do not lead us into temptation,*

> *But deliver us from the evil one.*
> *For Yours is the kingdom and the power and the glory forever. Amen.*
> (Matt. 6:9–13 NKJV)

Purpose: Ask the Lord to give you an opportunity to add significance to someone's life today. Watch for that opportunity. Ask God to use you this day for His intended purpose.

New!

Before Bed

Purpose: Ask yourself, "Did I live a life of purpose today?" What did you do to add value to someone else's life today? Commit to living a day of purpose tomorrow.

Prayer: Thank God for this day, asking Him to give you a restoring night's rest and a fresh start tomorrow. Thank Him for His steadfast love that never ceases and His mercies that are new every morning. Pray and confess the following Scripture out loud:

> *Who shall separate us from the love of Christ? Shall tribulation, or distress,*
> *or persecution, or famine, or nakedness, or peril, or sword? . . . Yet in all*
> *these things we are more than conquerors through Him who loved us. For*
> *I am persuaded that neither death nor life, nor angels nor principalities nor*
> *powers, nor things present nor things to come, nor height nor depth, nor any*
> *other created thing, shall be able to separate us from the love of God which*
> *is in Christ Jesus our Lord.* (Rom. 8:35, 37–39 NKJV)

Daily Tip: Be an agent of change in your life, the life of your family, the life of your church, the life of your organization, the life of your community and the life of your region.

Daily Notes:

_____

_____

_____

_____

_____

_____

_____

DAY 44

New!

Upon Waking

Prayer: Thank God because this is the day that the Lord has made. Rejoice and be glad in it. Thank Him for the breath in your lungs and the life in your body. Pray and confess the following scripture out loud:

> *He who dwells in the secret place of the Most High*
> *Shall abide under the shadow of the Almighty.*
> *I will say of the LORD, "He is my refuge and my fortress;*
> *My God, in Him I will trust."*
>
> *Surely He shall deliver me from the snare of the fowler*
> *And from the perilous pestilence.*
> *He shall cover me with His feathers,*
> *And under His wings I shall take refuge;*
> *His truth shall be my shield and buckler.*
> *I shall not be afraid of the terror by night,*
> *Nor of the arrow that flies by day,*
> *Nor of the pestilence that walks in darkness,*
> *Nor of the destruction that lays waste at noonday.*

A thousand may fall at my side,
And ten thousand at my right hand;
But it shall not come near me.
Only with my eyes shall I look,
And see the reward of the wicked.

Because I have made the LORD, who is my refuge,
Even the Most High, my dwelling place,
No evil shall befall me,
Nor shall any plague come near my dwelling;
For He shall give His angels charge over me,
To keep me in all my ways.
In their hands shall they bear me up,
Lest I dash my foot against a stone.
I shall tread upon the lion and the cobra,
The young lion and the serpent I shall trample underfoot.

Because I have set my love upon Him, therefore He will deliver me;
He will set me on high, because I have known His name.
I shall call upon Him, and He will answer me;
He will be with me in trouble;
He will deliver me and honor me.
With long life He will satisfy me,
And show me His salvation.
(Psalm 91 NKJV, in the first person)

New!

Before Bed

Prayer: Thank God for this day, asking Him to give you a restoring night's rest and a fresh start tomorrow. Thank Him for His steadfast love that never ceases and His mercies that are new every morning. Pray and confess the following Scripture out loud:

Love is patient, love is kind and is not jealous; loves does not brag and is not arrogant, does not act unbecomingly; it does not seek its own, is not provoked, does not take into account a wrong suffered, does not rejoice in unrighteousness, but rejoices with the truth; bears all things, believes all things, hopes all things, endures all things. Love never fails. (1 Cor. 13:4–8 NASB)

Daily Tip: A strong relationship with God comes through prayer and will help you understand His purpose for you.

Daily Notes:

_____

_____

_____

_____

_____

_____

_____

_____

DAY 45

New!

Upon Waking

Prayer: Thank God because this is the day that the Lord has made. Rejoice and be glad in it. Thank Him for the breath in your lungs and the life in your body. Pray and confess the following Scripture out loud:

I take up the whole armor of God, that I may be able to withstand in the evil day, and having done all, to stand. I stand therefore, having girded my waist with truth, having put on the breastplate of righteousness, and having shod my feet with the preparation of the gospel of peace; above all, taking the shield of faith with which I will be able to quench all the fiery

darts of the wicked one. And I take the helmet of salvation, and the sword
of the Spirit, which is the word of God; praying always with all prayer
and supplication in the Spirit, being watchful to this end with all perse-
verance and supplication for all the saints. (Eph. 6:13–18 NKJV, in the
first person)

New!

Before Bed

Prayer: Thank God for this day, asking Him to give you a restoring night's rest
and a fresh start tomorrow. Thank Him for His steadfast love that never ceases
and His mercies that are new every morning. Pray and confess the following
Scripture out loud:

Rejoice in the Lord always. Again I will say, rejoice! Let your gentleness be
known to all men. The Lord is at hand. Be anxious for nothing, but in every-
thing by prayer and supplication, with thanksgiving, let your requests be made
known to God; and the peace of God, which surpasses all understanding, will
guard your hearts and minds through Christ Jesus. Finally, brethren, whatever
things are true, whatever things are noble, whatever things are just, whatever
things are pure, whatever things are lovely, whatever things are of good report,
if there is any virtue and if there is anything praiseworthy—meditate on these
things. . . . Not that I speak in regard to need, for I have learned in whatever
state I am, to be content: I know how to be abased, and I know how to
abound. Everywhere and in all things I have learned both to be full and to be
hungry, both to abound and to suffer need. I can do all things through Christ
who strengthens me. . . . And my God shall supply all your need according to
His riches in glory by Christ Jesus. (Phil. 4:4–8, 11–13, 19 NKJV)

Daily Tip: Prayer is a discipline. Try to extend your prayer time by five minutes a day each week. This will help you to spend more time with God and
gives you a realistic goal.

Daily Notes:

_____

_____

_____

_____

_____

_____

_____

Day 46

New!

Upon Waking

Prayer: Thank God because this is the day that the Lord has made. Rejoice and be glad in it. Thank Him for the breath in your lungs and the life in your body. Pray and confess the following Scripture out loud:

> *Our Father in heaven,*
> *Hallowed be Your name.*
> *Your kingdom come.*
> *Your will be done*
> *On earth as it is in heaven.*
> *Give us this day our daily bread.*
> *And forgive us our debts,*
> *As we forgive our debtors.*
> *And do not lead us into temptation,*
> *But deliver us from the evil one.*
> *For Yours is the kingdom and the power and the glory forever. Amen.*
> (Matt. 6:9–13 NKJV)

New!

Before Bed

Prayer: Thank God for this day, asking Him to give you a restoring night's rest and a fresh start tomorrow. Thank Him for His steadfast love that never ceases and His mercies that are new every morning. Pray and confess the following Scripture out loud:

> *Who shall separate us from the love of Christ? Shall tribulation, or distress, or persecution, or famine, or nakedness, or peril, or sword? . . . Yet in all these things we are more than conquerors through Him who loved us. For I am persuaded that neither death nor life, nor angels nor principalities nor powers, nor things present nor things to come, nor height nor depth, nor any other created thing, shall be able to separate us from the love of God which is in Christ Jesus our Lord.* (Rom. 8:35, 37–39 NKJV)

Daily Tip: You are most effective when you use your gifts and abilities as a means to fulfilling your purpose.

Daily Notes:

_____

_____

_____

_____

_____

_____

_____

_____

Day 47 (Partial-Fast Day)

New!

Upon Waking

Prayer: Thank God because this is the day that the Lord has made. Rejoice and be glad in it. Thank Him for the breath in your lungs and the life in your body. Pray and confess the following Scripture out loud:

> *Is this not the fast that I have chosen:*
> *To loose the bonds of wickedness,*
> *To undo the heavy burdens,*
> *To let the oppressed go free,*
> *And that you break every yoke?*
> *Is it not to share your bread with the hungry,*
> *And that you bring to your house the poor who are cast out;*
> *When you see the naked, that you cover him,*
> *And not hide yourself from your own flesh?*
> *Then your light shall break forth like the morning,*
> *Your healing shall spring forth speedily,*
> *And your righteousness shall go before you;*
> *The glory of the LORD shall be your rear guard.*
> *Then you shall call, and the LORD will answer;*
> *You shall cry, and He will say, "Here I am."*
> *(Isa. 58:6–9 NKJV)*

New!

Before Bed

Prayer: Thank God for this day, asking Him to give you a restoring night's rest and a fresh start tomorrow. Thank Him for His steadfast love that never ceases and His mercies that are new every morning. Pray and confess the following Scripture out loud:

Is this not the fast that I have chosen:
To loose the bonds of wickedness,
To undo the heavy burdens,
To let the oppressed go free,
And that you break every yoke?
Is it not to share your bread with the hungry,
And that you bring to your house the poor who are cast out;
When you see the naked, that you cover him,
And not hide yourself from your own flesh?
Then your light shall break forth like the morning,
Your healing shall spring forth speedily,
And your righteousness shall go before you;
The glory of the LORD shall be your rear guard.
Then you shall call, and the LORD will answer;
You shall cry, and He will say, "Here I am."
(Isa. 58:6–9 NKJV)

Daily Tip: God created you and knows you (Ps. 139:13). His purpose for your life is perfect.

Daily Notes:

_____

_____

_____

_____

_____

_____

_____

_____

Day 48 (Day of Rest)

New!

Upon Waking

Prayer: Thank God because this is the day that the Lord has made. Rejoice and be glad in it. Thank Him for the breath in your lungs and the life in your body. Pray and confess the following Scripture out loud:

> *The Lord is my shepherd;*
> *I shall not want.*
> *He makes me to lie down in green pastures;*
> *He leads me beside the still waters.*
> *He restores my soul;*
> *He leads me in the paths of righteousness*
> *For His name's sake.*
> *Yea, though I walk through the valley of the shadow of death,*
> *I will fear no evil;*
> *For You are with me;*
> *Your rod and Your staff, they comfort me.*
>
> *You prepare a table before me in the presence of my enemies;*
> *You anoint my head with oil;*
> *My cup runs over.*
> *Surely goodness and mercy shall follow me*
> *All the days of my life;*
> *And I will dwell in the house of the Lord*
> *Forever.*
> (Psalm 23 NKJV)

New!

Before Bed

Prayer: Thank God for this day, asking Him to give you a restoring night's rest and a fresh start tomorrow. Thank Him for His steadfast love that never ceases and His mercies that are new every morning. Pray and confess the following Scripture out loud:

> The LORD is my shepherd;
> I shall not want.
> He makes me to lie down in green pastures;
> He leads me beside the still waters.
> He restores my soul;
> He leads me in the paths of righteousness
> For His name's sake.
> Yea, though I walk through the valley of the shadow of death,
> I will fear no evil;
> For You are with me;
> Your rod and Your staff, they comfort me.
>
> You prepare a table before me in the presence of my enemies;
> You anoint my head with oil;
> My cup runs over.
> Surely goodness and mercy shall follow me
> All the days of my life;
> And I will dwell in the house of the LORD
> Forever.
> (Psalm 23 NKJV)

Daily Tip: Your purpose indicates what you do with your life, and your talents help you to live out that purpose.

Daily Notes:

_____

_____

_____

_____

_____

Day 49

New!

Upon Waking

Prayer: Thank God because this is the day that the Lord has made. Rejoice and be glad in it. Thank Him for the breath in your lungs and the life in your body. Pray and confess the following Scripture out loud:

He who dwells in the secret place of the Most High
Shall abide under the shadow of the Almighty.
I will say of the LORD, "He is my refuge and my fortress;
My God, in Him I will trust."

Surely He shall deliver me from the snare of the fowler
And from the perilous pestilence.
He shall cover me with His feathers,
And under His wings I shall take refuge;
His truth shall be my shield and buckler.
I shall not be afraid of the terror by night,
Nor of the arrow that flies by day,
Nor of the pestilence that walks in darkness,
Nor of the destruction that lays waste at noonday.

A thousand may fall at my side,
And ten thousand at my right hand;
But it shall not come near me.
Only with my eyes shall I look,
And see the reward of the wicked.

Because I have made the LORD, who is my refuge,
Even the Most High, my dwelling place,
No evil shall befall me,
Nor shall any plague come near my dwelling;

For He shall give His angels charge over me,
To keep me in all my ways.
In their hands shall they bear me up,
Lest I dash my foot against a stone.
I shall tread upon the lion and the cobra,
The young lion and the serpent I shall trample underfoot.

Because I have set my love upon Him, therefore He will deliver me;
He will set me on high, because I have known His name.
I shall call upon Him, and He will answer me;
He will be with me in trouble;
He will deliver me and honor me.
With long life He will satisfy me,
And show me His salvation.
(Psalm 91 NKJV, in the first person)

New!
Before Bed

Prayer: Thank God for this day, asking Him to give you a restoring night's rest and a fresh start tomorrow. Thank Him for His steadfast love that never ceases and His mercies that are new every morning. Pray and confess the following scripture out loud:

> *Love is patient, love is kind and is not jealous; loves does not brag and is not arrogant, does not act unbecomingly; it does not seek its own, is not provoked, does not take into account a wrong suffered, does not rejoice in unrighteousness, but rejoices with the truth; bears all things, believes all things, hopes all things, endures all things. Love never fails.* (1 Cor. 13:4–8 NASB)

Daily Tip: The apostle John was known as "Old Camel Knees" because of the extensive time he spent kneeling in prayer. Prayer is a discipline. Try to extend your prayer time by five minutes a day each week. This will help you to spend more time with God and gives you a realistic goal.

Daily Notes:

_____

_____

_____

_____

_____

_____

_____

DAY 50: JUBILEE DAY

"Consecrate the fiftieth year and proclaim liberty throughout the land to all its inhabitants. It shall be a jubilee for you; each one of you is to return to his family property and each to his own clan" (Lev. 25:10 NIV).

"When the field is released in the Jubilee, it will become holy, like a field devoted to the LORD; it will become the property of the priests" (Lev. 27:21 NIV).

Jubilee Day in the 7 Weeks of Wellness is Day 50 of the program and is the day of celebration that ushers in the first day of subsequent cycles of 49-day "seasons" of your life. It is symbolic of overcoming and being set free, and it also signifies the continual offering of ourselves as living sacrifices, "holy unto the Lord" (as noted above in Lev. 27:21)—His possession.

> *The LORD bless you and keep you;*
> *The LORD make His face shine upon you,*
> *And be gracious to you;*
> *The LORD lift up His countenance upon you,*
> *And give you peace.*
> (Num. 6:24–26 NKJV)

Video Curriculum Questions

These questions are meant to be answered after watching the *7 Weeks of Wellness* DVD.

Introduction
What are some examples of the dietary and lifestyle elements presented in *The Great Physician's Rx for Health and Wellness* and *7 Weeks of Wellness DVD*?

_____

_____

_____

_____

_____

_____

Key #1
Scripture suggests boundaries that we can use to identify what God intended for us to eat. What are they?

_____

_____

_____

_____

_____

_____

_____

List a healthy substitute for each of the "dirty dozen" that Jordan discussed in the video.

_____

_____

_____

_____

_____

_____

_____

_____

_____

_____

Key #2

How can you identify an effective supplement?

_____

_____

_____

_____

_____

What are some key nutrients that we don't get enough in our regular diets?

_____

_____

_____

_____

_____

Key #3

What are the five major entry points for germs to enter your body? How often should you clean these during the day?

_____
_____
_____
_____
_____
_____
_____

What is "auto-inoculation"?

_____
_____
_____
_____
_____
_____
_____

Explain the primary ways that germs travel.

_____
_____
_____
_____
_____
_____

What percentage of the germs on your hands reside under your fingernails?

_____

_____

_____

_____

_____

_____

_____

_____

Key #4

What are the three major topics Jordan discusses in week 4?

_____

_____

_____

_____

_____

_____

_____

_____

Why is functional fitness so important?

_____

_____

_____

_____

_____

_____

What are some benefits of functional fitness?

_____

_____

_____

_____

_____

_____

_____

_____

What are three ways you can make movement more a part of your day?

_____

_____

_____

_____

_____

_____

_____

_____

Why are proper rest and sleep so important?

_____

_____

_____

_____

_____

_____

_____

Key #5

What types of toxins do we encounter daily?

_____

_____

_____

_____

_____

_____

_____

List some dangers of chlorine.

_____

_____

_____

_____

_____

_____

_____

What are two ways you can reduce household toxins?

_____

_____

_____

_____

_____

_____

Key #6
How can deadly emotions affect you physically?

_____
_____
_____
_____
_____
_____
_____
_____
_____

Consider who you need to forgive in your life. It might be a large offense or a very small one, but forgiveness is necessary. Without mentioning any names, tell someone you trust who you need to forgive in your life. Then ask your trusted friend to follow up with you in a week or two to see what progress you and the Lord have made in the area of forgiveness. Physically, forgiveness reduces your stress level and gives you a sense of control over the situation—allowing you to take responsibility for how you feel. Below write some steps that you can take to start your process of forgiveness.

_____
_____
_____
_____
_____
_____
_____
_____
_____
_____

Key #7

Discuss briefly what you believe God's purpose for your life is. What is it that you are uniquely gifted or positioned to do, and what steps are you taking to help fulfill that purpose?

_____

_____

_____

_____

_____

_____

_____

_____

Describe your passion, your personality, and your talents, and then tell how God has used those to fulfill your purpose in life. If you aren't yet sure what your gifts and talents are, pray daily for God to reveal the special plan and purpose he has for your life.

_____

_____

_____

_____

_____

_____

_____

_____

ABOUT THE AUTHOR

When Jordan Rubin was a nineteen-year-old college student, his body was attacked by a chronic, "incurable" digestive disease that affected his entire body. When conventional and alternative medical therapies failed, leaving him wheelchair-bound and at death's door, he looked to the Bible as a single, constant source for health and wellness. Today, at the age of thirty, he credits his victory over illness to an enduring faith in God and a revolutionary health program contained in the pages of *The Great Physician's Rx for Health and Wellness.*

Following his recovery, Jordan dedicated his life to transforming the health of others one life at a time. He earned the designation as a Doctor of Naturopathic Medicine from Peoples University of the Americas School of Natural Medicine, and more recently, earned a Ph.D. in Nutrition and Natural Therapies from the Academy of Natural Therapies. He is also a certified nutritional consultant, a certified personal fitness instructor, a certified nutrition specialist, and a member of the National Academy of Sports Medicine.

Prior to writing *The Great Physician's Rx for Health and Wellness,* Jordan authored *Patient Heal Thyself* (2003, Freedom Press) and *Restoring Your Digestive Health* (2003, Kensington Publishing). His most recent book, *The Maker's Diet* (2004, Siloam) has spent more than forty-two weeks on the *New York Times* Best Seller list (for Paperback Advice) since its release, and today there are more than 2 million copies in print. The success of *The Maker's Diet* prompted dozens of appearances on national TV programs and features in major newspapers and magazines.

In addition to sharing his message of good health, Jordan is the founder and chairman of Garden of Life, Inc., a health and wellness company based in West Palm Beach, Florida, that produces whole food nutritional supplements and personal care products. He is also president and CEO of Biblical Health,

Inc., a biblically-based health and wellness company providing educational resources, small group curriculum, functional foods, nutritional supplements, and wellness services.

He and his wife, Nicki, married in 1999 and are the parents of a toddler-aged son, Joshua. They make their home in Palm Beach Gardens, Florida.

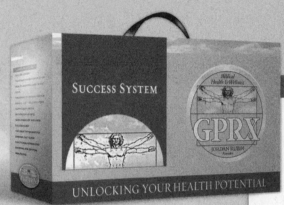
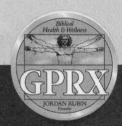

TAKING YOUR HEALTH
TO THE NEXT LEVEL

THE GPRX ULTIMATE SUCCESS SYSTEM INCLUDES ALL
THE EDUCATIONAL RESOURCES IN THE GPRX SUCCESS SYSTEM.
PLUS, YOU WILL RECEIVE WHOLE FOOD NUTRITIONALS AND
ADVANCED HYGIENE PRODUCTS DESIGNED BY JORDAN RUBIN
TO KICK START YOU ON YOUR JOURNEY TOWARDS
ABUNDANT HEALTH.

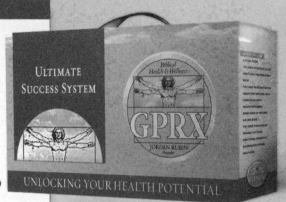

CONTENTS INCLUDE:

- The Great Physician's Rx for
  Health and Wellness Audio Book

- Seven Weeks of Wellness Video
  Curriculum *(with Facilitator's Guide)*

- Seven Weeks of Wellness
  Success Guide

- The Great Physician's Rx
  Dinning Out Guide

- Functional Fitness DVD

- Shopping for Optimal Health DVD

PLUS:

- Maker's Multi - *A Whole Food Vitamin and
  Mineral Formula*

- Omega-3 A.D. Cod Liver Oil Complex

- Super Greens - *Green Food and
  Vegetable Formula*

- Probio-Enzyme - *Probiotic and Digestive
  Enzyme Blend*

- Advanced Hygiene System

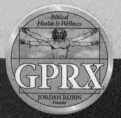

WWW.GREATPHYSICIANSRX.COM

INTRODUCING THE
BIBLICAL HEALTH INSTITUTE

FREE Biblically Based Introductory Courses on the Seven Keys to Unlock Your Health Potential

- In Depth Content on the Seven Keys

- The Latest Research on Nutritional Science

- 40 Hour "Biblical Health Coach" Certification Courses *(coming soon)*

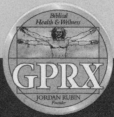

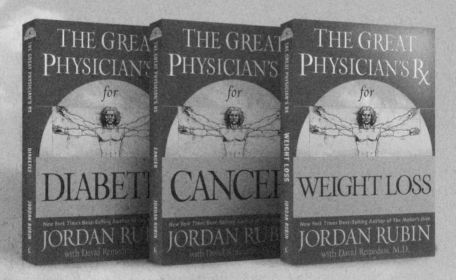
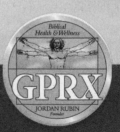

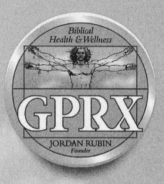